Acne Cure Clear Skin For Life

T0025174

strategies, medicine, and the body's inherent healing processes, not to replace the decisions you make with your medical professional.

Please take time to think critically.

Table of Contents

Acne Cure Clear Skin For Life

Introduction:

You wake up in the morning and dread to look in the mirror, only to find angry red inflamed zit/pimples situated on your face! You've tried everything from magic creams sold by infomercials endorsed by celebrities, prescription drugs and even worse, anti-antibiotics! Your depressed, hopeless and now think its in your genes or hereditary. Guess what? This couldn't be further from the truth, and in actual fact ANYONE can achieve clear skin!

Do not be bamboozled by the beauty/cosmetic industry selling their magic creams, they have conditioned society to think that acne is a normal part of life. Remember the beauty/cosmetic industry is worth over a billion dollars! They thrive on people's insecurity and conditioning innocent people with misinformation/inaccurate info.

In order to fix a any problem you must go to the root of it. In this case acne is a multi-faceted problem, however don't let this scare you. I will gladly break down ALL of the various causes and mechanisms in detail which trigger acne within our bodies.

If you are plagued by the curse of acne and believe that you are unable to control this chronic skin disease then this book is for you. In the following chapters you will come to an understanding of what truly causes acne and more importantly what you can do to solve and completely reverse this problem forever!

This book is not about pushing expensive pharmaceutical or

cosmetic products. In fact, the premise is that those may actually be exacerbating the problem, and wasting your hard earned money. Instead, in this book you will learn about how to treat acne at its root casual level rather than just at the symptomatic level. The whole concept is based on a holistic, scientific based and natural approach that shows that we have the ability to manage our own health if we treat our bodies with the respect, proper health strategies and elimination of food toxicity.

So what are you waiting for? Clear skin awaits you just turn the page!

Chapter 1: Uncovering the Truth

Acne is the eighth most commonly occurring disease in the world. It affects eighty to ninety percent of teenagers on the planet and for half of them, this chronic skin condition manifested by red and inflamed lesions lingers on until they are in their twenties or even their thirties. You have to realize the "common sense approach", if acne has been something assailing you ever since you could remember, let's say around age 11-13, then there is something you are doing on a chronic and long term basis every day to continually fuel the existence of this disfiguring condition.

If you are suffering from this chronic skin disease, or know someone who is, then the first thing you, or they, may have to tackle is your perception on this skin disease. It is common for people who are bearing the weight of this problem to feel lowered self esteem and even depression, but there are ways to deal with it and we will be looking at those in depth during the course of the next few chapters. This book does not offer a short term solution like so many of the so called pharmaceutical products that are on offered on the market. I suspect you may have tried some of these "miracle solutions" and quickly found that they did not match up to the hype or what was promised in the accompanying advertisement. With the disease affecting such a large amount of our society, there was no way that the big pharmacy companies were not going to try to make a buck by offering products purporting to wipe acne away virtually overnight.

Instead of proposing a miracle cure that tackles the

symptoms but not the causes, this book will delve into the problem more deeply and tackle it on a much broader front. We will look at what the causes are of the different types of acne and then show how to overcome the problem from a number of different angles including making changes to your diet and way of life.

From a medical point of view, the description for acne, goes something like this: "Acne vulgaris is a skin disease and condition that is characterized by red inflamed skin lesions, that occurs when hair follicles are clogged by mixture dead skin cells and an overproduction of sebaceous oils from sebaceous glands located in the skin." What that translates into for most victims is pimples, white heads, black heads (oxidized whiteheads) or a combination of the above. It is often accompanied by greasy/sticky sebum or oily skin and has a tendency of occurring on areas of the body where it is most visible and can cause the most embarrassment and even long term psychological damage. It is especially common among teenagers and adolescents as they go through changes in puberty and this can be a vulnerable age to find themselves confronting such a problem. This also accounts for the high levels of depression for teenagers suffering from acne. The teenager years are often fraught with anxiety and lack of self confidence and acne has the potential to add another layer to that difficult period.

First we must understand this problem is completely reversible! - That's right nobody, I repeat, absolutely nobody has to suffer from this disfiguring skin disease. We don't need these high powered chemical concoctions with dubious healing properties. All too often, we are told that acne is a heredity disease and that if we have it we are stuck with it. This couldn't be further from the truth, another favorite myth that all too often accompanies this problem is that it is as a result of unhygienic lifestyle habits. If that were true we would see acne being washed away with regular showers and any acne sufferer will tell you that that is not going to happen.

This amalgamation of myth, rumor and medical hocus pocus can easily leave victims feeling confused, depressed and hopeless. This book endeavors clear up the confusion, dispel the myths and offers practical solutions which if adhered to religiously will lead to change. It sets out to demonstrate that with a little education and some self discipline you can free yourself from the ravages of a very common skin disease that is not just the result of your genetic inheritance. You will learn the basic biochemistry of what is going on in your own body and understand what dietary changes can be made to overcome the root causes of this all too common skin complaint. Over the next few chapters you will learn that you are in charge of what is taking place in your body and you have the power to influence the outcome. In short, this is a book about hope and freedom for a misunderstood chronic skin disease that has ravaged a huge section of society at one stage or another, and has even caused suicide among people!

Did you know?....

Most cosmetic products you buy do nothing for your skin, but perhaps impact the superficial part of the skin temporarily, but if you want to rid yourself of acne permanently you need to go deep within. Did you know the products you are buying mostly contain fillers? Meaning that stuff you rub on your skin is made up of 95% water, waxes, oils, emulsifiers, preservatives, fragrances, and other chemicals that do not benefit your skin at all! Meaning for most products out there you are really buying over priced fillers, a brand, and these products have little to no effect on the long term for attaining healthy, clear and glowing skin.

Chapter 2: Futile Conventional Treatments

The treatment for acne legions has not really evolved over the last decade, and still till this day 99% of treatments fail to treat the underlying root cause but only treat the symptoms. One of the problems with acne is that because the disease is so widespread, there is a great deal of money to be made from sufferers desperate for some sort of relief from the problem. That does not mean that we are not seeing new products appearing on the shelves of the local supermarkets or drug stores, it just means that those that we are seeing are just rehashing the same failed medicines under different names. The base ingredients tend to remain the same. Meaning all your really receiving is marketing at its finest.

Here are some of the products that you can expect to find and the effects they will probably have. The name that they are traded under often changes so you may have to look keenly at the list of active ingredients on the deck to know exactly what it is that you are dealing with. Note: All these products treat the symptom and not the root cause.

Benzoyl peroxide: This one has been around a long time. It is comes in differing strengths (%5-10%) and is available as a soap, a gel or in one of several other lotion forms. Its main purpose is that it kills the active P. acne bacteria that is commonly found situated on your face. Remember bacteria is a secondary cause to the formation of acne, and P. acne bacteria thrive in anaerobic conditions causing the increased inflammation and multiplication of acne lesions.

How Benzoyl peroxide works? It uses oxygen molecules to intrude the breeding grounds of P.acne bacteria, and in short killing them and greatly reducing their numbers and spread, and completely dries out the pimple. The strategy of this over the counter product is kill off bacteria to eliminate acne to form or stop its existence. This happens as when oxygen molecules are introduced P. acne bacteria cannot thrive as they are multiply in anaerobic conditions, and thus they start to dwindle. Side effects known; it does cause dry skin and peeling that many acne sufferers will recognize, and it can go on to cause itching, stinging or even a rash.

Salicylic acid: Like benzoyl peroxide salicylic acid, which is derived from bark of the willow trees, this is mainly used as a wash for unclogging hair follicles that have become clogged due to build up of dead skin cells, sebum and keratin. It differs from benzoyl in that it does not kill active bacteria. However, it is used more as a peeling agent for clogged pores, and its main function is to allow dead skin cells slough off more easily. Both of these products are effective at unclogging pores but they do not solve the acne problem as their producers claim.

Sulfur creams: Sulfur creams are one of those products where you will probably have to look closely at the fine print to be aware that this is the active component. Because sulfur on its own has a bad smell, this product is almost always used in conjunction with other products which is one reason you will probably not find the word sulfur mentioned in the main product description. Its beneficial effects tend to be fairly limited other than drying out the skin during use and ceasing the spread of acne multiplication. It can cause rashes and irritation but may also cause skin discoloration which, in some people, may be quite severe. It can also lead to headaches and allergic reaction. Sulfur works by stopping the spread and propagation of P. acne bacteria, and again only treats acne at the symptomatic level.

Antibiotics: Perhaps one of the worst treatments for acne, in many fields the use of antibiotics is beginning to prove controversial and this is also the case when using them to treat acne which is what some doctors will do. Overuse of, and misuse of antibiotics is starting to have some unforeseen effects both on individuals and in the ecosystem. There can be no doubt that these products have played a vitally important role in modern medicine but their overuse is beginning to see the development of resistant bacteria and that could have massive repercussions. One of their disadvantages is that they tend to be non selective and though they are good at killing bacteria that we don't want, such as that that is linked to acne, they often kill other vital bacteria, specifically in our gut known as the microbiome, at the same time we are slowly discovering that much of the bacteria in our bodies is crucial to our health! For this reason we need to think very carefully before utilizing products that offer short term gain, but which may provoke health problems of a different nature that often times are far worse somewhere further down the road in life.

Accutane: This product was first trialed as an acne treatment in 1979. It is a derivative of vitamin A. Initially it was hailed as the silver bullet for acne problems and a miracle drug for acne suffers. It has had some good results as far as acne is concerned, but its use is becoming more controversial as we learn more about its long term side effects. Because it is a systemic drug its effects are far from limited to targeted areas.- It effects our whole body! Here is a brief list of the side effects of Accutane which often times can be long term; hair loss, vision problems blindness, Crohn's disease, Colitis, headaches and reduced blood flow to the brain.

I personally am an x-Accutane user and can advocate and

vouch for the extreme toxicity of this systemic drug I experienced. In essence this drug is an oral pill, and works by drying out the oil glands within your body, and it's by no means selective, meaning it targets all of your oil glands throughout your body! I personally started having bowel movement troubles (extreme constipation) during my second course of Accutane and stopped immediately, fortunately my digestive health healed over time (6-8 months), but after that I learned my lesson and never went back to pharmaceutical drugs.

This drug is extremely taxing on the liver due to the fact that Accutane really is an overdose of vitamin A, fat soluble vitamin, meaning it gets stored in your liver. Note: ***DO NOT*** overdose on vitamin A supplements the effects can be just as bad. With a little knowledge, you are in a far better position to understand what it is that the pharmaceutical industry is offering even if they do not necessarily include the main active ingredient in the name of the product that they are selling. You will have a better idea of the possible risks and understand that these products target the symptoms rather than the root causes. As you can tell by now the pharmaceutical approaches only strives to mask symptoms or artificially induce physiological responses from the body which are not at all natural. The premise of this book is our body is an intelligent design, and simply needs the right environment and materials to function optimally.

Unfortunately the pharmaceutical companies are not the only ones to have spotted a lucrative gap in the acne treatment market. The cosmetic and beauty industries have also climbed onto the bandwagon. If the pharmaceutical companies were unable to address the root causes it does not take too much imagination to see that cosmetic companies are going to be even less likely to do so. Most of the products offered by the cosmetic industry are designed to either camouflage the problem or are cleansers with some supposedly near miraculous healing properties. It is understandable that from time to time a person suffering from acne would want to hide the symptoms. When doing so, however, they need to be aware that whilst they may camouflage the problem in the short term, they risk aggravating it over the longer term.

Make up as a whole, creates a layer over the skin that is not natural. I am sure that any suggestions to give up make up will only fall on deaf ears, but victims of acne need to achieve some middle ground. Don't wear makeup except on those occasions when it is absolutely necessary and between times get the makeup off and leave the skin clear so that it is exposed to natural air (oxygenation) as nature intended. This will at least give your skin an opportunity to recover a little. After an occasion when makeup has been worn the skin should be cleaned as soon as possible and as thoroughly as possible. There are few things that are going to add to your acne problems quicker than leaving the skin covered with cheap makeup over night. When choosing a cleanser do some research and do not simply believe what the cosmetic industry tells you about the miraculous effects of its cleansers. I recommend natural witch hazel as an astringent for use.

Acne is a problem that stems from within the body and most pharmaceutical products treat only the external symptoms whilst cosmetic solutions may actually compound to the problem by further blocking pores. I don't want this to lead to a sort of helpless feeling or depression. Acne is completely reversible and the truth is anyone can acquire clear skin naturally without spending thousands of dollars at esthetician, futile cosmetic products or pharmaceutical drugs. This book is here to empower you the reader to take control of your acne condition regardless of its severity.

Ultimately this book is here to help you in incremental step to achieve clear skin for life! Lets dive into the case study in the next chapter shall we?

Chapter 3: The Kitava Case Study & Sugar

Let's now pop across the ocean to the tiny island of Kitava in the Pacific. This difficult to reach island, uncorrupted by the western influence, with its tiny population is one of the few places in the world not to have not assimilated the Western diet. In 1989 a doctor by the name of Staffan Lindeberg went there to examine the health of the people and what he discovered was quite extraordinary. Amongst the general population that Dr. Lindeberg was accustomed to working with he would expect to see acne levels at between 79 and 95 percent in adolescents. Among the adolescents on Kitava the acne rate was zero to nonexistent! The doctor was intrigued by such a sharp difference and he immediately set about trying to find what it was that was so different about these islanders that exempted them from the ravages of acne. In the end the main difference he found was their diet! The Kitavans lived entirely on a natural diet that was made up mainly whole foods; fish, fresh vegetables, eggs, fruit and coconuts. Fruits do contain natural sugars, loaded with fiber and other phtyonutrients which compensate for harmful effects sugar.

Back in America researchers are now seeing reductions in acne levels amongst people who consume a diet high in whole foods such as fresh vegetables, organic lean meats and low in dairy. It is thought that dairy, being high in hormones may lead to acne. One hormone often associated with acne is called androgen which is a male hormone that seems to cause acne in both men and women and is also linked to excess body hair in women. Androgen hormones seems to increase with excess insulin production, and insulin spikes when excess levels of sugar are found within our blood stream.

The Kitava diet is all natural and foods contain plenty of omega 3,6, 9 (fish and coconut), fiber, and the whole range of vitamins and trace minerals from both fruits and cruciferous vegetables.

What is interesting is when the western diet was incorporated into the Kitavan lifestyle, guess what? Acne started to appear! Isn't this incredible? This validates a few things, one acne's primary influence is based on what we eat or to be more specific what we absorb through the consumption of foods. Number two, acne is a completely reversible chronic skin disease if we make the appropriate lifestyle changes. Earlier in the introduction of this book I spoke about the "common sense approach", and discussed if acne has been persistent all your life, common sense dictates there must be something you are doing perpetually wrong all your life for this condition to continue. In this case, it's what you eat!

Now there is more complexity to the acne condition, and as I promised this book will give you the full in depth understanding of acne. But above is a foundational principle on which to operate on, and there are other factors as well which contribute to acne, so keep reading. I want to give you the full insights so you can have an understanding and be empowered!

We need to accept that our bodies are like machines and that if we use the incorrect fuel we run the risk of having problems at some stage down the road. In terms of our diet, the modern, so called, Western diet has changed dramatically over the past two hundred years and most dramatically over the last fifty years. Over the last decades humans have learned to manipulate carbohydrates, grains, etc to increase its shelf life at a price. What is that price? High glycemic (GI) indexed ranked foods that are almost instantly digested by our bodies and readily convert into sugar for fuel, and contain little to no nutrients. Fiber, essential fats, trace minerals, and vitamins are all stripped from the majority of processed foods we eat, and this includes fast, junk foods as well.

Glycemic index (GI) - This is a index that measures how quickly foods are broken down, rapidly converting them into glucose (sugar) within the blood stream. Note; high ranked GI foods tend to be fast, junk and processed foods! Whole natural foods are typically considered low ranked GI foods. Whole foods contain; fiber, nutrients, vitamins, trace minerals, etc. While high GI foods are devoid of everything, hence why they readily convert into glucose once digested. The correlation between acne and high GI ranked food is quite intriguing, and an upcoming chart in this chapter will describe the correlation between the two.

By far the biggest change to our diet has been the introduction of refined sugar. The amount of sugar that we consume has shot up, and continues to do so despite the fact that purchases of refined sugar in supermarkets has actually gone down. The reason for the continuing climb in sugar intake is that almost all foods found in our local supermarkets have been added with one form of sugar or another. We need to be "proficient label readers" as sugar is disguised under many names under the ingredient decks, here is a list of different types of sugar you may come across, maltose, dextrose, sucrose, glucose, fructose, high fructose corn syrup (HFC contains traces mercury!), cane syrup and inulin to name a few.

Two hundred years ago sugar played a tiny part in the average person's diet. As an imported luxury it was something that was only consumed on special occasions. After a while sugar production was expanded to meet the "sweet tooth" cravings of society and lucrative potential at the marketplace. The price went down whilst availability went up. The average American today consumes twelve and a half teaspoons of sugar per day whilst the World Health Organization recommends that we should only be consuming half that much. That translates to one hundred pounds of sugar per person per year which is up from four pounds per person per year in the 1700s.

The affects on our health have been astronomic. Instead of a continuing rise in life span we are now starting to see a fall as people succumb to many modern health problems, chronic degenerative diseases, such as type 2 diabetes and obesity. So what does all this have to this sugar have to do with acne? Well believe it or not there is a strong correlation between intake of refined sugar and acne. Dermatologist are slowly coming to the awareness of this fact and the role diet plays with acne.

Since we are on the subject of sugar/high GI ranked foods and its effects on exasperating acne I want to give you a brief prelude of the chapter in this book " Different Types of Acne". I will extrapolate the main points of focus and show you the relation to sugar/high GI ranked foods and acne. Take a look down at the chart below how sugar/high GI foods influence acne..

High GI FOODS > Spike insulin levels secretion > Releases(insulin like growth factor) IGF1- growth hormone > Promotes excess secretion of sticky and oxidized sebum > Rapid uncontrolled skin cell division> Sebum and mixture of (malformed)dead skin cells clog within pores > P.bacteria feed on the blockage and multiply> Defensive response of white blood cells ensues (inflammation) and then acne forms.

For your knowledge see below 4 categories of acne:

Red inflamed acne/zit = classic acne

White head = uninfected comedo

Black head = oxidized sebum, basically a white head but oxidized.

Cystic acne = typically fueled by excess androgen hormones, and appear deep within the skin. It can be thought of as an exaggeration of the classical acne.

Chronic disease states are merely nothing more than the expression of perpetual bodily breakdown , which as a result defensive repair and response mechanisms activate and cause the various visible symptoms we see today, categorized as "chronic diseases", and in this case acne. Symptoms are really messages notifying us that the operating machinery is out of order and gone awry. The body is a perfect design, intelligent, self-sufficient and extremely economical. Acne can be thought to be as the harbinger of more imminent chronic disease states.

Today it is difficult to avoid sugar if you rely on fast food, industrially altered food or canned drinks. Big food corporations have managed to add sugar, in its many differing forms, to just about any product they make.

Our diets have become very high in carbohydrates and we must understand that carbs are really just sugar under a different guise. Nearly all pastries and cookies will contain sugar, and so will things like whole wheat bread, thus where possible you will need to vastly reduce the amount of carbohydrate you eat. Once again this is most easily done by eating whole food. A good replacement for bread would be natural brown rice or quinoa, these are minimally processed foods and are a far better alternative to bread. Remember to uptake your cruciferous vegetables.

We should not really be surprised that the link between acne and what we eat is so strong. Acne is a health problem and we cannot really expect to have optimum health on a poor diet. Cutting out sugar, caloric restriction, reducing carbs dramatically and switching to drinking good old fashioned water may be all that is required to end your acne problem. It is also recommended you supplement for any nutritional deficiencies, we will discuss this later in the book. It is certainly a good place to start and is the only one mentioned so far in this book that treats the cause rather than the symptoms. There is no big money to be made from encouraging you to eat healthy whole food and drink lots of water so don't expect this message to get the push that pharmaceutical, dermatologist and cosmetic companies can give to their products either.

Food Elimination Diary

In this sub section I would like to give you completely free cost effective strategy to assist in you in the remission of acne and get to the final goal of clear skin. I am pretty sure we've all heard of diaries right? But in this case this is not an ordinary diary, but in fact this is a food diary, and the way it works is simple.

You pick one food and consume them one at a time and record them in your food diary, and slowly implement other foods one by one, in doing so you are watching for foods that aggravate or flare up your acne. It should be done in weekly intervals, and you basically choose one food wait a week, and see what happens. If it causes you acne then eliminate it, and move on to something else until you can find something that settles with your body, most likely natural foods.

The aforementioned information in the chapter saves you the trouble and eliminates a lot of food right from the get go. So rule of thumb, NO fast , refined, processed or junk foods! This diary is extremely helpful for people who may have adverse effects to eating things like almonds, and other natural whole foods. Usually, if this occurs it means your body has some sort of malabsoprtion or processing issue, and in many cases its fat malabsoportion. It is recommend you supplement 1200mg of lecithin for any fat malabsoprtion issues. - Remember everyone is different although our biochemistry basically functions the same, some foods may cause an acne flare up in person A, but not person B. So, observe for food intolerances, digestive issues and even bowel movements that are difficult, and see what happens.

Chapter 4: Different Types of Acne

Androgenic acne:

This acne is notorious and affects both men and women in their teens, twenties to fifties and is hormonal related. This type of acne is also responsible for the disfiguring cystic acne. Typically found in the T-zone and singular pimple/zit. Red and inflamed, if it is a whitehead it is not infected. Androgenic acne is Influenced by DHT/ IGF1-growth factor creates excess sticky (oxidized sebum). This type of acne is a hyperproliferation causing problem, excess and uncontrolled cell division/growth. Due to lack of nutrition, vitamin, minerals and especially food toxicity, cells in the pores divide very rapidly causing a blockage.

How processed foods, junk foods and refined foods trigger a chain reaction of acne inducing biochemistry (simplified) **High GI FOODS > Spike insulin levels secretion > Releases IGF1- growth hormone > Promotes excess secretion of sticky and oxidized sebum > Rapid uncontrolled skin cell division> Sebum and mixture of (malformed)dead skin cells clog within pores > P. acne bacteria feed on the blockage and multiply> Defensive response of white blood cells ensues (inflammation) and the acne forms**.

Note: Squalane makes up approximately 12% of sebum, and it is this substance that oxidizes (damages) and is extremely comedogenic. The oxidation of squalane occurs due to presence of free radicals which in short, molecules (found within cells) that are incomplete -they're missing electrons!

Thus in order to become stable they steal electrons from the nearest oxygen molecule, and ergo this cascading effect repeats itself. This means compromised and damaged oxygen molecules are rampant within the body, and thus oxidize components which they make up, sebum (squalane).

The lack of anti-oxidants within the body (due to malnutrition) to counter act the effects of oxidization is one of the many primary causes of inflamed skin lesions, acne. Remember bacteria is a secondary cause to the formation of acne, and P. bacteria thrive in anaerobic conditions, ergo when oxygen molecules lose their electrons (due to free radicals from unhealthy foods) they are no longer stable, less oxygen present, ergo this creates perfect breeding grounds for the spread of P.bacteria which then causes a mediated response from the immune system signaling antibodies to clean up the excess propagation of P.bacteria, which then causes RED inflamed acne. Proper oxygenation is essential for glowing and robust skin, and is often overlooked.

As we can see the lack of anti-oxidants found in foods and compromised molecules due to food toxicity significantly contribute to the formation of acne directly, and the correlation between free radicals and anaerobic conditions due to food toxicity (junk food, processed, high sugar) which influences androgenic acne and its formation is quite evident. Thus, the importance of eating anti-oxidant rich foods! (Natural green leafy vegetables & fruits!)

Nutritional Solution For Androgenic Acne :

-Keep DHT (testosterone) regulated. Keep IGF-1 growth factor (insulin) regulated.

- Zinc Deficiency: Take zinc picolinate 50mg daily scientifically proven anti-inflammatory effect on skin lesions and sugar control.

-Herb Turmeric: Anti-inflammatory effect - take it as a tea.

-Omega 6 fatty acid: Will have a liquefying affect on sebum

-Omega 3 fatty acid: Anti-inflammatory effect

-Deficiency in Vitamin A: Vitamin A(10,000 - 20,000 IU): Stabilizing effect on cells within the follicle that divide. DHT inhibition

- Vitamin B5: Sugar control, helps with processing fats and oils.

-Beta sitosterol: DHT Inhibition

-Saw palmetto: DHT inhibition

-Chromium: Blood Sugar stabilizing effect

-Vanadium: Blood sugar stabilizing effect

-Magnesium: Multi functional mineral

-Vitamin C: Anti inflammatory, stabilizing benefits and assists in proper growth

ELIMINTAE FROM DIET : DAIRY, JUNK FOODS, PROCESSED FOODS, REFINED FOODS, ANY FOODS THAT RANKS HIGH GI(glycemic index), FOODS HIGH IN CARBOHDRYATES

-Intake more whole foods, lean meats, vegetables, etc

-Topical Treatments: Retina A (retinol), ACV (apple cider vinegar), Witch Hazel.

Before reaching for some chemical that will treat the symptoms let's take a deeper look at some nutritional options that could save you a great deal of money and bring about many health benefits and at the same time reverse your acne. The first thing you will want to do is knock out those insulin spikes that we have seen in the preceding chapter. This will strengthen your body's immune system whilst at the same time lowering the production of androgen hormones. Reducing dairy will also help as it is high in hormones. Zinc deficiency is common with this type of acne.

The herb Turmeric has a further anti inflammatory effect and can be made into an herbal tea, which should be drunk twice a day.

Omega 3 oils are also anti inflammatory, whilst Omega 6 thins the oils that are causing the follicles to get blocked. Vitamins A, B5 and C will all help in your fight, vitamin A is of particular importance as it will help stabilize skin cell division as well as speeding the skin's capacity to repair itself. Vitamin C over immune system boost and body health, and B5 for sugar control and inhibition excessive of sebum oil.

Saw palmetto and Beta sitosterol will help keep down levels of Dihydrotestoserone-alpha (DHT) which disrupts brain signals and can cause acne development. Saw palmetto an herb extract and is made from the fruit of the saw palm. It is good at preventing testosterone which can go on to form harmful DHT. Be careful with this herb, as this one in particular may cause adverse effects you'll want to talk to your general practitioner or local herbalist before doing any of these strategies.

Chromium helps reduce insulin resistance and is available in broccoli, green beans as well as beef and poultry.

Vanadium is a micronutrient believed to help stabilize blood sugar which we have seen is so important. It is found in dill, eggs and pepper.

Magnesium deficiency can lead to inflammation. It is an essential mineral that can often be found in low supply within the body. Too much can be toxic so avoid supplements and instead increase your intake of green leafy vegetables, legumes, nuts and whole grains.

Hydrochloric Acid (HCL) is naturally produced in the stomach and it is frequently deficient. It can be supplemented with Trikatu which is a common ayurvedic medicine and it encourages HCL production by the body.

This may all sound very complicated, but all of the dietary deficiencies here can be tackled if we move away from fast food and processed food and adapt to a natural diet that is high in vegetables, low in dairy and contains plenty of protein. Remember to keep carb intake low and virtually eliminate added sugar in any form.

As a topical treatment you may want to try Retina A which is vitamin A derivative, and is great for revitalizing the skin. Washing with apple cider vinegar (ACV) restores acidity to the skin and creates a protective layer that helps prevent further infection. Dilute this very cheap product before use. It can simply be diluted with water and used on a cotton wipe. Witch hazel is another natural ingredient that is good for removing excess oils from the skin and is an active ingredient in many face washes.

Adrenal Acne - Stress Acne:

Symptoms/Causes: similar to androgenic acne.

Nutritional Solution:

-Keep sugar and caffeine intake low. Keep blood sugar stable.

-Same vitamins, minerals and fats as androgenic acne.

-Take probiotics.

- Increase lean meats/ protein

- Vegetables

 -Natural Sea salt; Usually if your craving salt it could mean your adrenal glands are deficient in salt.

Topical Treatments:

Salicylic acid & Glycolic acid

Zinc oxide creams

Commonly referred to as stress acne, adrenal acne bears a lot of similarities to androgenic acne in the way that it presents itself but it is often accompanied by loss of sleep and other anxiety indicators. The oily skin faced appearance is produced by the hormone cortisol in combination with a diet high in sugar and carbs. Other than on the face there will be few pimples produced. There will be, however, high levels of oil on the face.

Both sugar and caffeine will add to the production of stress hormone cortisol, and these should be eliminated from the diet wherever possible. Instead eat plenty of protein and leafy green vegetables. As with androgenic acne the same vitamins will be of help as will be consumption of probiotics & fermented foods such as Sauer kraut.

Salicylic acid used as a cleanser is a useful exfoliant which will help decrease the oily excretion and assist in the sloughing off of dead skin cells. Glycolic acid, a naturally occurring substance, is often included in skin care products that will rejuvenate skin without aggravating it.

Zinc oxide cream provides a skin barrier and this allows skin to heal.

How to differentiate Adrenal acne from Androgenic acne? Answer: Skin is very oil, has a few pimples, but face is mostly covered in oil as oppose to androgenic acne where face is covered in a lot of singular pimples.

One thing that will confirm that you have adrenal gland problems will be a craving for salt. Adding sea salt to your diet will help improve the functioning of this gland. (adrenal gland)

Digestive Acne:

Symptoms/Causes:

-Rash like acne covering from forehead, cheeks and chin

-Immune system induced acne

-Problem processing: starches (sugar)

-Dysbiosis in the gut

-Low stomach acid

Nutritional Solutions:

Eliminate:

-Gluten, Grains, Legumes, Egg and Dairy.

- ANYTHING found in a box with a high shelf life.

-ANY food intolerances.

Add/Consume:

- Fermented foods

-Bone soup

-Gelatin

-Mushrooms

-Algae

-Glutamine powder /supplements

-ACV (internal)

-HCL supplements

-Food elimination diary + Fasting

-Reduce calorie intake

 -Take probiotics

Additional Advise:

-Keep sugar and caffeine intake low. Keep blood sugar stable.

-Increase protein, fat, and more cruciferous vegetables.

-Same vitamins, minerals and fats as androgenic acne.

-Take probiotics.

- Lean meats

- Natural sea salt. -Usually if your craving salt it could mean your adrenal glands are deficient in salt.

Topical Treatments:

N/A This is a deep rooted internal issue, thus treating it from a topical approach is futile. Although you are more than welcome to use retina- A and Salicylic acid to treat current existing acne. As soon as you start correcting your digestive problems you'll see this type of acne disappear and reverse almost instantly.

This particular acne manifests in a rash like manner often occurring on the forehead and face. It is normally related to problems in the digestive system and these very often relate back to problems with sugar processing and low levels of stomach acid.

Removing dairy, eggs, gluten and grains is the most effective way to reduce this problem as these are the foods that are most likely to generate intolerance that triggers the acne. Fermented foods will increase gut bacteria as will yoghurt which, although a dairy product, is a great bacteria supplement.

Fat intake can be increased without adding to the carb intake by consuming bone broth which will also increase your body's intake of gelatine.

Once again you can use good old apple cider vinegar but in this case as a toxin flush. Two tablespoons of ACV added to a glass of warm water and drunk twice a day will do wonders. It is advisable to rinse out your mouth after drinking ACV as the acid can damage the enamel on your teeth. Low stomach acid is common in this form of acne and it can be increased through hydrochloric acid (HCL) supplements. Algae supplements can be taken in a tablet form but the dampened tablet can also be rubbed against the infected areas.

Glutamine supplements increase the availability of amino acid to the body which in turn increase the health of the digestive system. At the same time it lowers the desire for acne promoting sugar.

Calorie reduction can also benefit this particular type of acne. You will probably find that calorie intake will go down automatically simply through the changes to the diet recommended here, but to reinforce that you may want to consider a light intermittent fasting regime which will give the dysfunctional digestive system time to recover.

Liver Acne:

Signs/Causes:

-Body is burden and overloaded with toxicity, stemming from adrenal, androgenic and digestive acne!

-Combination of different components of the body, involving food toxicity, excess hormones (by products), blood sugar issues - dysglycemia.

-Liver acne takes longer periods of time to develop.

-Lymphatic system is clogged.

-Liver acne is found on neck, back, shoulders

Nutritional Solutions:

-Probiotics

-Fasting --liver will detoxify itself

-Citrus natural drinks

-Vitamin C

-Vitamin E

-Lecithin

-Vitamin A

-Bile salts

- Selenium

-Zinc

-Magnesium

-Milk Thistle

-Glutamine supplement

This acne is seen mostly on the back, shoulders and neck and is often aggravated by some of the other acne that we have seen already. It manifests itself when the body is overloaded with toxins and hormones which we have seen are present in other forms of acne. The liver is the body's main filter system (detox organ) and is therefore prone to creating this skin health problem when it becomes overloaded.

Probiotics help the body deal with some of the toxins it is carrying by boosting the beneficial bacteria levels, strengthening the microbiome. Probiotics are found in fermented foods and yoghurts (Unsweetened). To further address the buildup of toxins in the liver short spells of intermittent fasting (16 to 36 hours) will allow the liver to rid itself of toxins and this can be further supplemented by drinking green and herbal teas, natural citrus drinks like lemon tea and that old favorite, water.

Lecithin is an easily available food supplement that should be taken with food. It is excellent in increasing absorption of fatty acid which helps the liver get back to optimum efficiency levels. Bile salts help to flush impurities from the liver which further raise optimum liver function. Milk thistle is a great method to increase bile production.

Mineral additives including selenium, zinc and magnesium will all benefit this condition.

Topical Treatment:

Again for the same reasons as digestive acne you will need to treat yourself from within.

Thyroid Acne:

Signs/Causes:

Combination of dry and oily skin

When cortisol (stress hormone) is perpetually produced this causes the thyroid to slow down! This is a compensatory measure taken when cortisol levels remain elevated. Thus, the thyroid is slowing down in response to the adrenal gland secreting constant cortisol. Now the skin becomes dry due to the thyroid gland slowing down.

Oily skin equates to excess oil and dry skin equates to lack of moisture, not lack of oil. Thus, putting a cream to "cover it up" does not really create moisture or moisturize it. The skin posses its own moisture factors, and the problem is underneath not on the surface! Ergo, working on fixing the digestive system & blood sugar system will indirectly affect the thyroid gland. --Again, the entire human body is linked and we need to view it as a unified "system" and not in separate components. (The medical model and pharmaceutical industry treats the body as a separate components, treating symptoms only.)

When you continually apply moisturizing creams you are suppressing your skins own moisture factors causing you to buy more, more and more of it! Creating a cascading downward spiral effect on your skin.

Fun Fact: What is in your moisturizer? **Answer:** Most likely water, wax, preservatives, emulsifier , fragrance, and oil. - These are all fillers, and most products only contain anywhere between 1%-2% active ingredients.

Tell me does anything you see on this general ingredient deck for moisturizers appear to be healthy and worth your hard earned money? NO! Remember to achieve glowing clear skin; your body is your temple and whatever you put inside it will manifest outwardly on your skin too!

For some strange reason people believe rubbing a "magic" cream on their skin for moisturizing somehow helps us, but in actual fact we are just feeling the product on the superficial surface level! - It just masks the underlying problem.

Nutritional Solutions:

-Probiotics

-Fasting

-Glutamine supplements

Bone soup (anything that helps build cartilage)

-Stabilize blood sugar levels: Vitamin B5, B-complex, Vanadium, Cinnamon, Chromium,

-Controlling oily skin : Vitamin B5 higher doses

-Stay away from unhealthy foods; refined, processed, fast foods

Note: Remember your thyroid gland is responsive to its biochemical surrounding meaning, if it is exposed to a toxic environment, consequences follow. By treating the body holistically the thyroid will also be affected, and when applying nutritional strategies, elimination of food toxicity, and even slow deep breathing for oxygenation the thyroid will revert back to its healthy state. Unless there is an autoimmune problem or some other mechanical issue.

Topical Treatments:

-Vitamin C creams

- Vitamin B5 creams

Thyroid acne is commonly referred to as dry acne this is one of the most complex forms of acne. When that cortisol level remains too high it can cause the thyroid to over compensate by slowing down and this results in the opposite affect and thus the dry acne effect. There is a common tendency to apply creams to this problem in the hope of re-moisturizing the skin. As we have seen so often in this book, the problem runs far more deeply than just the symptom and adding creams just enhances the problem. The cause of the dryness is internal and that needs to be addressed or the problem will simply continue. The source of a healthy glow to your skin needs to come from being totally healthy inside and not just from some product coated on externally.

Once again probiotics will help as will glutamine supplements. Bone soup will increase fat intake and help by adding to cartilage. It is crucial to bring blood sugar level down and eliminate spikes and this will be done by following the basic diet we have already mentioned, and also incorporating intermittent fasting. Extra vitamins such as B5 and B complex also have a stabilizing effect. Vanadium and chromium supplements should be taken and cinnamon based teas will bring further benefits.

Glutamine supplements restore healthy gut and digestive systems and this, as always, this is crucial to skin health. Bone soups will add cartilage and healthy fat to the system.

The thyroid is always an indicator of unhealthy surroundings brought about through body toxins. Any measure that lowers the level of toxins entering the body will have beneficial effects.

You will find that the use of vitamin C and B5 creams will speed recovery up.

Premenstrual Acne 2 types: Progesterone & Estrogen:

Sign/Causes

-Progesterone hormone similar to androgenic acne flare ups: singular lesions, whiteheads, inflamed and red.

-Occurs during that "time of the month" near day 21-28.

-Estrogen/metabolites estrogenic hormones cause bumps on the jaw line

Nutritional Solution Progesterone Acne:

-Similar approach to androgenic acne

-Zinc Picoloinate

-Vitamin A

-Soy product

-Bio-flavinoids

-Fermented soy products

-Vitamin E

-Selenium

-Phytoestrogen (plant based products)

Topical Treatments:

Retinoid A creams

Nutritional Solution Estrogen Acne:

-Probiotics

-Fat metabolizing supplements

-Selenium

-Zinc

-B -complex

- Vitamin B5

-Broccoli

-Cauliflower

-Cabbage

-Calcium D glucorate

-Increase fiber intake from whole foods!

-Flaxseeds

-Kombucha

-Eliminate fast foods, refined, processed etc

Topical Treatments:

Retina A & Progesterone creams

There are two types of acne that are specific to women and they both relate to hormone activity. The first is progesterone and the second is estrogen related.

Progesterone acne occurs at the approach of the monthly period and looks very much like androgenic acne. It produces spots, whiteheads and individual lesions. It can be treated in much the same way as androgenic acne including the application of Retinoid A skin cream.

Estrogen acne has a particular distinction in that it causes bumps along the jaw line. Consume probiotics and fat metabolizing supplements as well as selenium, zinc, vitamin B and B 5 supplements. Include plenty of broccoli and cauliflower in the diet as well as flax seeds and Kombucha. Increased fiber intake will be beneficial but you should get enough of this if you increase your intake of whole foods and do away with fast food and industrially processed food. Soy products, including fermented soy, have been shown to reduce the amounts of estrogens in the body and obviously this is beneficial to overcoming this acne. Phytoestrogens are commonly found in many plants including soy, chick peas and legumes as well as nuts and seeds. Adding these to the diet will therefore help elevate estrogens to more balanced levels.

As you will have seen by now there is a great deal of overlap in the way that all these different types of acne are treated, and much of it comes down to common sense changes to your diet. These strategies are not going to bring any benefits to the pharmaceutical industry and so it is not in their interest to promote them. The changes are probably something that you recognize as being the right thing to do, but now acne has now given an added motivation, so use it. The benefits of eating natural whole food on which we evolved will go far beyond just reversing your acne.

It is unfortunate that we live in a world where so much of what we do is driven by money. You are obviously free to purchase expensive drugs or beauty products as you please, but they will only touch the outer layer of the skin called the epidermis. Beneath that is the dermis and lower still is the subcutaneous layer and by simply treating the epidermis you do not even touch the deeper layers. That needs to be done from within in a holistic manner if you are to truly overcome this chronic skin condition.

Chapter 5: Formation of Acne Differantion Process

It is important that we understand that the primary cause of excess division of skin cells is as a result of high Glycemic index (GI) food. These are foods that have a higher than normal impact of blood sugar levels and obviously includes all types of added sugars.

The skin is the largest organ of the body and the most visible so it makes sense to understand a little bit about it, especially if we are suffering from skin problems. The skin performs some incredibly important functions which we take very much for granted. Skin cells that we see actually started out far deeper in the layers of skin and they make their way upwards, where they eventually become skin as we know it. The outer layer of cells that are our visible skin become more filled with keratin as they rise up toward the surface where they are actually no longer living cells but are now hardened specks made up of protein.

The whole process is somewhat complicated but what we need to understand is that during the process any biochemical or structural problems will result in defects in the cells. What we see as zits or pimples near the surface of the skin, is in fact the result of some dysfunction in the cells that will have started much earlier in the process than when we actually see the visible symptoms. Any problems or defects in cell division or structure are exacerbated when we consume excess sugar. It acts as a kind of accelerant to the problem so lowering the blood sugar levels is always going to produce benefits in terms of the health of our skin. We have already looked at ways to do that and will do so in more depth in the next chapter.

There are many factors that affect the cells as they make their way up through the layers of skin to their final position on the very surface. The skin cells themselves produce bio-chemicals and the way in which they do this is very dependent on the availability of the correct fats and vitamins. The most important of these is Vitamin A because this particular vitamin plays a crucial part in the construction of cell structure. Whilst many of the vitamins we have mentioned play important supporting roles in the overall health of our skins, it is Vitamin A that is the primary building block of skin nutrient and therefore overall skin health.

Understanding the importance of Vitamin A in regards to the skin is very important. It is an underlying factor in skin health issue. There are different ways of ensuring that we get the correct amount of Vitamin A to support healthy skin. The first way is to address any deficiencies through eating the appropriate foods that will supply this vitamin and the second is through taking supplements. Supplements is a sure way to ensure that you are getting a sufficient supply of this vitamins, so you can start by taking vitamin A 10- 20 000 iu per day in a supplementary form. At the same time you should be upping your intake of those naturally occurring sources of Vitamin A such as sweet potatoes, carrots, meats, leafy green vegetables and winter squash.

It should be noted that Vitamin A is best absorbed when in partnership with Vitamin D3 and so you want the two in combination in order to achieve the best results. Vitamin D3 is known as the sun shine vitamin, most of us get enough of this particular vitamin through sunlight exposure but if you are living in an area deprived of sunlight you can easily up your intake through consumption of eggs, oily fish, mushrooms and liver.

One other method of absorbing Vitamin A is as a cream applied directly to the affected skin. Retinoic acid can only be taken only with a prescription from your dermatologist or doctor. It comes in strengths that range from 0.25 to 0.1 percent depending on the area of the body that it is needed. A gentler version that requires no prescription is called retinol. It is far less potent that its' prescribed counterpart Retinoic acid and so you will need to apply it at higher concentrations of between 2% and 5% percent.

Chapter 6: Solution

I hope that by now you have read enough to realize that acne and all its associated problems such as black heads, white heads, cyst and excess oily skin excretions stem from internal problems rather than just the surface skin issues. It is natural to want to attack the most visual manifestation of the problem, but attacking the symptoms is going to provide temporary relief at the very best. In many cases it will not even do that. Instead the whole issue has to be tackled holistically starting with what you put into your body in the first place.

Whilst this may seem glaringly obvious many of us have lost track of what a healthy diet consists of, thanks largely to the food industries ability to advertise its industrially altered products as having health benefits where none actually exist. Big industry takes food and processes it in large quantities. They then require that it has an increased shelf life or additional flavor in order to replace the taste that is knocked out of it during the factory process. There are many chemicals that they add in order to do this including colorants, fillers, and artificial flavors. There are three substances they use in large quantities in nearly all industrial processing that is really bad for our health. These are salt, trans fats and sugars.

They all come in a wide range of different disguises and there are hundreds of different ways of describing sugar alone. One way of avoiding these additives is to become an expert at deciphering the fine print on food labels but as soon as you eat anything that has been altered at the industrial level you are going to find it extremely difficult to avoid them. Rule of thumb for food if it has a long ingredient deck or you cannot pronounce the ingredient, you should avoid it. Avoid anything in a found in a box.

Sugar, be it in the form of cane sugar, palm sugar, high fructose corn syrup or one of the many other versions is very difficult to avoid. Sugar is the major product that our bodies have not evolved to deal with and it is this area that is creating the most chronic health problems, including acne. Our high blood sugar levels are very often the source of our skin problems and it is therefore imperative that we get our sugar levels stabilized. We can spend hours squinting at labels trying to do this, or we can opt for the more sensible route of eating whole and unprocessed foods.

Upping our intake of fresh vegetables, meat and fish will have a dramatic effect on the health of our skin. We need to get hold of a Glycemic Index (GI) chart and this will quickly give us a handle on those foods that we should be avoiding. It is quite amazing when you discover what foods have high GI levels and therefore add to our rising blood sugar levels. One of the major reasons that the big food corporations have managed to get such a grip on the food market is that of convenience. They have recognized that people are often time pressed and that they would rather eat a pre cooked meal that only needs thirty seconds in a microwave rather than go to the trouble of cooking for themselves. All of us need to examine this issue in terms of our overall health. It is true that preparing meals from raw ingredients is more time consuming, but are we going to allow that to let us spiral into a life of obesity, diabetes and acne problems (to name but a few) or are we going to take control of what goes into our bodies and enjoy better health? We all need to fall in love with the cooking process again and with the advent of the internet we are never far from recipes that are both healthy and can be prepared in just minutes.

Anything we put into our bodies is going to affect our skin positively or adversely. This obviously also translates to smoking and abuse of alcohol or drugs. You do not need to be a skin specialist to understand that these things will translate into poor skin health.

Once we have adapted to a healthier diet and have taken control over what goes in, then the next obvious step is to reverse the state of toxicity our bodies' have built up. Once more there is no need for rocket science or a medical degree here. Eating healthy, exercise and lots of pure water is going to go a long way, and have a plethora of positive effects, and especially promote vital, glowing and clear skin.

Diet Template:

1. Salmon, mackerel, and any other fatty fish that is an excellent source of omega 3, 6 & (sea food is highly recommended see the Kitava case study).

2. Fruits and vegetables such as carrots, apricots, and sweet potatoes

3. Spinach, kale, cabbage, broccoli and other dark green and leafy vegetables.

4. Tomatoes.

5. Brown rice --moderation is key, too much brown rice can still spike insulin level in blood stream.

6. Quinoa - preferred over brown rice.

7. Turkey or chicken breasts- organic.

8. Pumpkin seeds, flax seeds, almonds, sunflower seeds -- excellent sources of vitamin E. Again, moderation is key as excess amounts tends to break certain people out.

9. - Probiotics; Fermented Foods - Sauerkraut, Kombucha, Miso, Pickles.

10. Juicing your vegetables and fruits at home is a great option too! Use your own juicer.

11. Caloric restriction, important note: Do not snack throughout the day. I found my acne's influence stemmed from binge eating like habits throughout the day, which in my case exasperated my androgenic acne by increasing insulin production. Restrict yourself to eating when your ONLY hungry, not because you're bored or for a sugar rush.

I would strongly suggest you only eat 1-2 times throughout the day. No eating in between. I personally don't eat past 7pm.

12. Fasting is one of the most cost effective and FREE easy to use strategies to assist in ridding yourself of acne. There have been well documented cases of people fasting and literally clearing their acne in a matter of days (usually 5- 14 days). How it works? In this day and age we are constantly eating, not only constantly eating, but OVEREATING. When we "fast" we put a halt to our bodies' digestive processes of which is taxing, and we give opportunity for our body to rest and recover. Especially if you're eating high GI ranked foods, fasting is a effective way to get rid of the food toxicity accumulated within our bodies.

Don't believe main stream media and their façade with acne. Acne in truth, is simply a manifestation of internal distress which manifest outwardly as skin lesions. Whether, hormones, foods, etc, these all play a crucial component to the existence of acne. The old adage is true, you are what you eat, to be more specific you are what you absorb!

Ashley's Personal Supplement Regiment:

Wild Alaskan Salmon Fish Oil - 1,000mg (180 EPA/ 120 DHA) - anti inflammation

Beatine HCL - 500mg - Increases strength of digestive process , stronger absorption

Chromium and Vanadium- 125mcg - Blood sugar stabilizing effect

Vitamin E - 1,000IU - Protects the oxidization (damage) of sebum oils

Astragalus - 500mg - Drives the penetration of other supplements further in the body/cells

Pro-biotics - Acidophilus Bifidus 6 billion active cells - Strengthening our microbiome

Niacin (B3 buy the flush free or time release kind) - 500mg - Assists with sugar processing

L-optizinc with copper - 30mg (take two capsules a day)- Assists with sugar processing & anti inflammation

-Magnesium - 500mg - multi-functional purpose

-Vitamin A - 10,000-20,000 IU - DHT inhibition and normalizes expression of skin cell division

Vitamin D3 - 3,000 - 5,000 IU - most effective in combination with vitamin A.

 -Vitamin B5 - 500 - 1,000mg - Assists with sugar metabolizing

-Saw Palmetto with flax and pumpkin oils - 160mg (for androgenic acne only) - DHT inhibition

-Vitamin C - 1,000mg - 3,000mg a day - Overall immune boost, mutli-functional purpose

* If you feel this is a little too overwhelming to keep track of you can always look into taking good quality multivitamin drink (powdered) supplement that contains all the above dietary supplements. -Just mix with water. I personally do both.

Ashley's Personal Acne Story:

I suffered from every type of chronic skin problem you can think of. Acne is a problem I have struggled with ever since I can remember. It all began at the age of 11 and I suffered with it for over a decade! There were days, I felt hideous, unwanted, and just plain ugly. I remember crying myself to sleep and having such low self-esteem feeling helpless, hopeless and cursed.

I tried it all myself, miracle creams, toxic oral medications, antibiotics and even spent thousands of dollars at estheticians for laser acne therapy. Trust me I can tell you from my personal experiences that these are all a waste of time and your hard earned money! I've spent countless occasion in the dermatologist's office being prescribed rehashed brand name pharmaceutical drugs, nothing ever seem to change apart from the brand name. When I brought up the possibility of diet and the correlation to acne, this notion was always immediately dismissed instantly, and of course I believed the professional authoritative figure at the time because they know what's best, right? WRONG!

After countless attempts to do things the futile conventional way, the wrong way, I became so frustrated and thought I should just give up. And, I almost did, but I decided I would start doing my own research for myself and take a different approach. Fortunately living in the information age where info is almost instantly available on any given subject matter, I started to dive into in depth research, and learn the truth, the FACTS about acne. I realized if I wanted to conquer this problem I had to have a better understanding of physiology, biochemistry, skin, diet, nutrition and of course acne.

I joined countless online forums, watched ample videos, lectures and read a bunch of scientific articles. Slowly, but surely progress was being made and revealed to me was the truth behind acne. Like a jig-saw puzzle coming together in perfect congruence, so was my understanding of acne, the picture started to surface in perfect clarity and I was one step closer to acquiring the clear skin we all covet for.

I realized I was being lied to, not only me, but society was being feed misinformation in regards to acne. Most programs or treatments out there on the net are futile and only mask the symptoms of acne without actually treating the root cause. I started to see how the financial greed of a few created this misinformation, and pushed treatments and product to helpless and innocent individuals like you and me. I am not trying to go all conspiracy theory on you, but acne is such a lucrative market and business, so why would these "experts" ever want to cure this chronic skin condition?

We've all seen these infomercials of celebrity endorsed products claiming how they cleared their skin, these are all false and misleading long term solutions. Nothing more than a marketing ploy to entice people into buying their products. I also began to see how little these skin experts (including my dermatologist) knew about the complex and dynamic nature of the skin. They barely get taught the nutritional side of things, and it seems they are almost always trained to push pharmaceutical products only.

What I found really was a broken system that did not really care for the people, but only cared for profit margins of huge corporations. This is so anti-humanity on so many levels, and to compound to the problem a lot of times more often than none, these conventional treatments exasperate the problem and make it even worse!

I started to find more natural and nutritional roads to heal my chronic skin condition. I started viewing the skin as an organ and the need to treat it from within, and not fixing my problems by relying on some magic concoction smothered on my skin. I learned about the various layers of the skin, biochemistry, skin cells, and the multifaceted roles of nutrition, deficiencies and malnutrition.

I realized how EASY it was to reverse every single type of acne condition anyone suffers from. No one, I repeat no one has to suffer from acne, and the good news is that it is so easy to reverse. You can start seeing clear skin within weeks by following the above mentioned nutritional and supplementary protocols, and obviously eliminating certain food toxicities and intolerances. I broke down the complexity of the nature of acne in the most simplest of forms, and addressed the various types of acne. All you have to do is identify the symptoms with the descriptions I provide for each type of acne and find out which type you struggle with. I did ALL the guess work for you. (-It's possible you can suffer from a combination of acne types.) - The good thing is a lot of these nutritional strategies overlap.

Then follow the instructions outline to the letter and start seeing results within 2 weeks time! I cannot guarantee a time frame for clear skin because everyone is at a different stage when it comes to acne and the amount of toxicity you have exposed and burdened the body with, and the life style you have lived. But what I can tell you is that you will see significant results!

For me personally, I suffered from every type of acne on the list, believe it or not. But by far one of the most painful and psychologically traumatizing types was androgenic, cystic acne. My biggest problem at the time was trying to figure out why my skin condition persisted? I used the "common sense approach", and I thought to myself if my acne is still flaring up this is my body's way of notifying me something is not right. I soon found out that although I was eliminating fast foods, junk foods, and processed foods, there was still an underlying trigger causing my cystic acne to exists.

What was the problem? Refined carbs! Pasta, breads and noodles, these were foods that were disguised as "healthy foods", but in reality are considered refined carbohydrates and instantly converted into sugar in the blood stream for fuel(high GI ranked foods). This epiphany or revelation whatever you want to call it was the pivotal point of change in my life. I realized all my life I let these seemingly appearing and marketed healthy foods infiltrated my diet, and these were indeed the foods causing the perpetual chronic skin condition I suffered from.

I quickly replaced those toxic food choices with more wholesome foods, such as quinoa, green leafy vegetables, flax seeds, lean organic meats etc. Guess what? My cystic acne dramatically decreased, and reverted to normal size manageable acne and its severity was lessened. Now the silver bullet is when I started adding dietary supplements I aforementioned (I was deficient in many vitamins and minerals), and within 3-4 weeks I acquired clear, sustainable, healthy and glowing skin! Soon my friends started asking me what exactly was I using, and I simply told them I just changed my diet up and started supplementing. They were in disbelief!

I am a testament that clear skin can be achieved without spending thousands of dollars. Stop listening to the mainstream lies and start becoming empowered by doing your own research, following my scientifically proven steps, and change your life style according to the template I have provided. I can ensure you it will make a significant impact on your skin health, and you really have nothing to lose. Rest assure acne is not some hereditary curse you have to live with for the rest of your life, as a matter of fact, it's more of an environmental and lifestyle influenced chronic skin condition as discussed earlier and proved with abundant evidence.

I would also suggest you look up the glycemic index provided below. Note: Do not even attempt to use dairy despite the low ranking, it is filled with hormones that influence androgenic and other types of acne. (from my personal experience)

Glycemic Index Basic Template

Low GI (<55), Medium (55-61), High (70>)

Vegetables

Asparagus 15

Broccoli 15

Celery 15

Cucumber 15

Lettuce 15

Peppers 15

Spinach 15

Tomatoes 15

Chickpeas 33

Cooked Carrots 39

Fruits

Grapefruits 25

Apple 38

Peach 42

Orange 44

Grape 46

Banana 54

Mango 56

Pineapple 66

Watermelon 72

Dairy

Plain Yoghurt 14

Soy Milk 30

Skim Milk 32

Whole Milk 27

Ice Cream 61

Protein

Peanut 21

Dried Beans 40

Lentils 41

Chickpeas 47

Lima Beans 46

Pinto Beans 55

Black Eyed Beans 59

Chapter 7: Bonus Natural Remedies

I am assuming that you have now bought into the concept of improving your health from the inside out. As an added bonus here are some natural remedies that will supplement the process and won't require huge expenditure.

Cinnamon powder: Cinnamon tea helps to balance blood sugar levels and lower testosterone. You can either steep a cinnamon stick in boiling water for fifteen minutes or add a half teaspoon of ground cinnamon to boiling water and allow to steep. Don't take more than half a teaspoon per day.

Turmeric mask: Mix two table spoons of ground oats, one teaspoon of turmeric, three tablespoons of yoghurt and a few drops of honey. Apply to the affected area and leave on for fifteen minutes. Rinse afterwards.

Green tea spray: Green tea inhibits sebum production and also has anti bacterial properties. Simply brew up a cup full of this tea and then either spray it on or apply it with a cotton ball twice per day.

Baking soda facial: Mix a paste with three teaspoons of baking soda then mix it to form a fine paste. It makes a great exfoliate with added anti fungal properties.

Aloe vera and honey mask: Aloe vera has been used to heal skin problems due to its soothing properties. Take a stem of the aloe and squeeze as much juice as you can into a bowl. This will leave you with a slightly desiccated leaf, but you can get further gel from within by cutting open the leaf and scraping out the interior contents. Mix in four drops of lemon juice and one tablespoon of honey then stir together. Apply to the affected area for twenty minutes then rinse with warm water.

Aspirin face mask: Another method for a simple but effective mask is simply to mix a crushed, uncoated aspirin with water and coat the area to be treated for twenty minutes.

Baking soda /coconut oil mask: This has anti bacterial properties from the coconut oil and a drying agent in the baking soda. Mix one teaspoon of baking powder and one teaspoon of coconut oil. Apply generously.

Steam: Steam is a great way to open pores and allow impurities to be flushed out. All you need is a large bowl of boiling water then as soon as the steam becomes cool enough to bear place a towel over your head and the bowl and remain there for fifteen minutes which will generate a good sweat. After that wash your face well.

Linen hygiene: It is a good idea to wash your pillowcase and sheets at least once a week to reduce the chance of re-infecting yourself from bacteria.

Resist the urge to touch: It is very easy to succumb to the urge to touch, scratch or squeeze your acne. This can risk permanent scarring, so you want to avoid this.

Whilst all of these natural remedies will prove useful and inexpensive I hope that you will see them as extra additions to the need to treat the problem from within rather than as cures in themselves.

Conclusion:

The main message you need to take away from this book is that you have the power to change your skin. You are not a helpless victim of genetics or unsanitary lifestyle, but can master your own destiny and all without the aid of expensive cosmetic products or harmful drugs. The whole process of healing relates to taking a holistic approach to the way that you treat your body. This will help you overcome the acne problem you face, but will also address other health issues of which acne may be just a precursor to. The underlying issues to acne are as follows; food toxicity (fast, junk, processed & refined) & intolerances, malnutrition, malabsoprtion and vitamin deficiencies. These elements influence all the "different types of acne" mentioned earlier in this book.

The skin is a delicate organ that is a billboard for what is going on with your overall bodily health. It can be thought as the window to your overall health. You can have it healthy and glowing if you pay attention to what you eat and drink, get some exercise and just a touch of sunlight. Now is the time to take control of your health.

The skin contains many layers, and current skin treatments only treats superficial aspect of acne, first layer of the skin. Many sheets/layer of skin are found underneath and by only treating the superficial exterior by celebrity endorsed skin creams we are really doing both our bodies and our skin a disservice. The problem is found deep within! - Although there are surface superficial skin problems like contact irritation etc, but most skin problems are from within and will manifest outwardly from chronic toxicity.

These alternative health strategies is what the beauty/cosmetic industry do not tell you about! Not only are these strategies beneficial to your whole biological system (body), but they are so much more cost efficient and effective!

You would save thousands of dollars if you applied these strategies into your daily routine, you will notice the results of clear skin, vitality and longevity through these strategies. Why burns your hard earn money on skin treatments that simply don't work?

The premise here is simple, and that is the body is an intelligent design, extremely economical and only needs the right raw materials to function at optimum efficiency. I think by now you have realized the hereditary myth of acne is debunked, and in reality you are in control of every facet of your life in regards to good health. Acne is not a randomly occurring disease, but chronic, long term and is a symptom of underlying issues that have occurred over an extended period of time. It can be thought to be like a harbinger of more imminent chronic degenerative disease states.

With all the empowering information I have provided you with I am sure you will see clear skin in no time. Remember all the guess work has been done for you! You just have to identify what type of acne you have and follow the right protocol. That's it, it's simple.

Take control of your health and beauty by empowering yourself with this knowledge and applying what you have learnt. You won't regret it.

I am Ashley Dawnson, an advocate of good health, vitality, longevity and ultimately quality of life. The medical model's approach never made sense to me, whether it was in regards to other chronic degenerative diseases states or acne. I found the solution to my acne through nutritional roads, and these healthy alternative strategies just make more sense.

I was inspired to write this book out of the struggles, pain and personal experiences of my life, and I truly hope it has impacted you in a positive way to help you gain your confidence back, and of course clear your skin! As promised I delivered a book with no gimmicks, facts and ultimately the truth about acne, I am sure it will significantly help you. I got tired of seeing mean spirited cosmetic companies preying on insecure people who struggle with acne and using them as a cash cows by selling them futile products to make a quick buck.

I really wanted to make a difference and it seemed there were no true long term viable solutions out there. I made it my mission to inform and share this knowledge with YOU and acne suffers across the globe!

It never made sense to me to poison the body, mask symptoms, or knocking out inherent bodily functions to forcefully produce results. We need to become critical thinkers and question the standards of today. Wishing you all the best in your journey to clear skin! :)

If you found this book helpful would you be kind enough to leave a quality review on Amazon? Thanks! Please see the LINK below..

LINK: http://amzn.to/2ro7cfi

Other recommended books for better overall health:

Weight Loss http://amzn.to/2nodZ7e Author Jenifer Cruz

Yoga http://amzn.to/2ovn6n3   Author Pamela Maverick

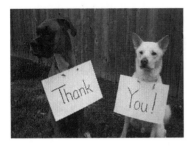